Simple Guide

to

the Chakras

Susie Newman

ISBN 978-1-4303-1399-1

I would like to thank all my trusted friends and family for their support in helping me to complete the book.

Just imagine in your mind's eye

the calm sea within

the quiet harbour of the heart

and in the distance

there is a sunset full of love, hope

and promise.

If only we take the time to listen to our heart

then we are always guided home to the

Harbour of the Heart…..

Harbour of the Heart

Within the Harbour of the Heart

resides the beginning and the start

to love and to be loved

is all we can do to make sure

that it becomes true.

Every moment we take the journey

to discover our true worth and

to become the lover

and the beloved will be the key.

Each day that dawns this life does form

as we venture forth to create

our Destiny…

CONTENTS

Chapter One

THE SEVEN CHAKRAS

Personal Energy Field

We all have our own personal energy field and this is known as the Aura. It is not visible to the naked eye and yet it plays a vital role linking the mind, body and spirit.

The Aura is similar to an egg-shape and acts as an electro-magnetic field encircling the body.

The Aura consists of seven subtle bodies containing the physical, emotional, mental, spiritual, astral, etheric and super etheric bodies. It often absorbs negative and positive energy therefore it is important to maintain a healthy Aura.

CHAKRAS

The chakras are wheels of energy that are linked to our personal energy field the Aura. The chakras connect the three subtle bodies and these are known as the mental, emotional and spiritual bodies.

There are seven chakras altogether starting at the base of the spine gradually move upwards from the Base chakra, Sacral chakra, Solar Plexus, Heart chakra, Throat chakra, Third eye and finally to the Crown chakra.

Chakras are energy centres that continually open and close similar to the petals on a rose. The chakras are able to absorb and radiate different colours of light transforming it into energy.

They are made up of particles of light that vibrate at different levels and take in and give out the life force energy therefore it is extremely important that they are in good working order.

When there is an even flow of energy a person will feel in harmony and balance. When there is an uneven flow of energy the chakra will become blocked and will influence a person's energy levels and well-being. These chakras are a direct indication of how we are feeling at any given moment.

BASE CHAKRA

The Base chakra is located at the base of the spine and is the colour red. It has 4 petals and is associated with the element of earth. This chakra is also known as the root chakra that connects and supports us in the material world, by giving us a sense of security.

When this chakra is in balance we will feel grounded and able to bring our ideas into action. When this chakra is out of balance we may feel angry, aggressive and out of control. This disconnection from the earth can leave us feeling light-headed and disorientated. When the life force energy is not flowing through this chakra it becomes blocked and we are just concerned with everyday survival and may miss out on the joys of life.

Colour: Red

Located: Base of the Spine

Number of petals: 4

Element: Earth

Gemstone: Red Jasper

Balanced: Ability to survive in a material world and bring ideas into action

Unbalanced: Angry, aggressive, and ungrounded

SACRAL CHAKRA

The Sacral chakra is located a few inches below the navel and is the colour orange. It has 6 petals and is associated with the element of water. The Sacral chakra connects us to our creative energy, sexuality and vitality for life.

When this chakra is in balance there is an abundance of creative energy that we can connect to. When this chakra is unbalanced we are no longer able to go with the flow of life and we may feel exhausted and low in energy.

When the life force energy is blocked there will be difficulty in maintaining sexual relationships and we may feel fearful.

Colour: Orange

Located: few inches below the Navel

Number of petals: 6

Element: Water

Gemstone: Carnelian

Balanced: Abundance of creative energy

Unbalanced: Low vitality and exhaustion

SOLAR PLEXUS CHAKRA

The Solar Plexus chakra is located above the navel and is the colour yellow. It has 10 petals and is associated with the element of fire. This chakra connects us with our personal power and helps us to develop our self-confidence.

When this chakra is in balance we are able to act on our intuition and gut reaction. When this chakra is unbalanced we are no longer centred and may feel anxious or nervous with low self-esteem.

When the life force energy in this chakra is blocked we are unable to hold our personal power and we may feel low in energy and lack self confidence.

Colour: Yellow

Located: above the Navel

Number of petals: 10

Element: Fire

Gemstone: Calcite or Citrine

Balanced: Personal power and self-confidence

Unbalanced: Anxious and lacking in self-esteem

HEART CHAKRA

The Heart chakra is located in the centre of the chest area and is the colour green. It has 12 petals and is associated with the element of air. When the Heart chakra is in balance and open we can give and receive unconditional love.

We will experience humility and feelings of compassion for others and ourselves. When this chakra is unbalanced we may become controlling, manipulative and arrogant.

When the life force energy is blocked in the Heart chakra we may experience domineering, arrogance and selfish attributes. When the life force energy is flowing we may experience love for ourselves and others, forgiveness and acceptance.

Colour: Green

Located: Chest area

Number of petals: 12

Element: Air

Gemstone: Aventurine or Rose Quartz

Balanced: Compassion and unconditional love

Unbalanced: Control and unable to give and receive love

THROAT CHAKRA

The Throat chakra is located in the throat area and is the colour blue. It has 16 petals and is associated with the element of sound. This chakra is connected to how we communicate with others and our ability to express ourselves to the outside world.

When this chakra is in balance we can speak freely and openly to others. When this chakra is unbalanced we may have a fear of speaking our truth and unable to discuss our thoughts and feelings.

When the life force energy is blocked we will be unable to express how we feel or think. When it is unblocked we are able to discuss our feelings enabling us to project our voices resulting in the ability for the energy to flow.

Colour: Blue

Located: Throat area

Number of petals: 16

Element: Sound

Gemstone: Sodalite or Sapphire

Balanced: Able to communicate & express oneself

Unbalanced: Unable to speak our truth with others

THIRD EYE CHAKRA

The Third Eye chakra is located in the centre of the brow and is the colour indigo. It has 2 petals and is associated with the element of light.

This chakra connects us to our visions and dreams and when open gives us the ability to perceive other realms of reality.

When this chakra is in balance we are able to follow our intuition and have clear visions of where we are going in our life. When this chakra is unbalanced we are unable to have clarity and may feel unclear about our future.

Colour: Indigo

Located: Centre of the forehead

Number of petals: 2

Element: Light

Gemstone: Lapis Lazuli

Balanced: Vision and dreams

Unbalanced: Unable to see clearly and lack of imagination

CROWN CHAKRA

The Crown chakra is located at the top of the head and is pure white in colour. It has 1000 petals and is associated with the element of thought. This chakra is our connection to the divine source and the divine light.

When this chakra is in balance we will feel guided by the divine force and have a personal connection to our own inner light.

When this chakra is unbalanced we may feel depressed, frustrated and disconnected from our higher self.

You may find that by having this area massaged it will help the life force energy to flow properly or you could wear hats or scarves to protect this area.

Colour: White

Located: Top of the Head area

Number of petals: 1000

Element: Thought

Gemstone: Clear Quartz or Amethyst

Balanced: Connected to the Divine

Unbalanced: Depressed and isolated

Chapter Two

3 MINUTE SIMPLE MEDITATIONS

Meditations are a way of clearing our daily stresses and distracting thoughts that we may experience and accumulate throughout the day.

It often helps to still the mind thus bringing tranquility and peace so that we may focus on one specific idea or thought form.

The use of colours and gemstones can balance the seven chakras and bring the equilibrium back into one's life.

3 minute meditation Silver Shower of Light

When you take a shower in the morning or evening this meditation will help you to focus on positive energy to have that feel good factor.

Our personal energy field often records and stores positive and negative thoughts, memories and emotions. Therefore it is important to purify and cleanse the Aura on a daily basis.

1. Place yourself under the shower and visualize a silver shower of light that pours over your head and covers your whole body.

2. Imagine the silver shower of light flowing over your body as it lifts your spirits and cleanses any negative energy.

3. Now, perceive yourself pulsating with a silver positive energy.

3 minute meditation for the Base Chakra

1. Close your eyes and take 3 deep breaths as you breathe out on the last breath bring your attention to the base of the spine and imagine the Base chakra as a red flower.

2. Now breathe in the red hue and see this being absorbed by the flower until it has completely saturated the area.

Imagine the energy going deep into the earth, grounding and stabilizing you.

3. Once you have completed this exercise take another 3 deep breaths and open your eyes.

3 minute meditation for the Sacral Chakra

1. Close your eyes and take 3 deep breaths as you breathe out on the last breath bring your attention to the area just below the navel and imagine the Sacral chakra as an orange flower.

2. Now breathe in the orange hue and see this being absorbed by the flower until it has completely saturated the area.

Imagine the vibrant colour revitalizing your creative energy and allowing the life force energy to flow through you.

3. Once you have completed this exercise take 3 deep breaths and open your eyes.

3 minute meditation for the Solar Plexus

1. Close your eyes and take 3 deep breaths as you breathe out on the last breath bring your attention to a few inches above the navel and imagine the Solar Plexus as a yellow flower.

2. Now breathe in the yellow hue and see this being absorbed by the flower until it has completely saturated the area.

Imagine the vibrant shade covering this area leaving you feeling centred and confident.

3. Once you have completed this exercise take 3 deep breaths and open your eyes.

3 minute meditation for the Heart Chakra

1. Close your eyes and take 3 deep breaths as you breathe out on the last breath bring your attention to the centre of the chest area and imagine the Heart chakra as a green flower.

2. Now breathe in the green hue and see this being absorbed by the flower until it has completely saturated the area.

Visualize the petals of the flower slowly opening and closing for you to give and receive love.

3. Once you have completed this exercise take 3 deep breaths and open your eyes.

3 minute meditation for the Throat Chakra

1. Close your eyes and take 3 deep breaths as you exhale on the last breath bring your attention to the throat area and imagine the Throat chakra as a blue flower.

2. Now breathe in the blue hue and see this being absorbed by the flower until it has completely saturated the area.

Now sing the word 'ah' and let the sound resonate around you. Imagine that you are speaking clearly and expressing yourself to others.

3. Once you have completed this exercise take 3 deep breaths and open your eyes.

3 minute meditation for the Third Eye Chakra

1. Close your eyes and take 3 deep breaths as you exhale on the last breath bring your attention to centre of your brow and imagine the Third Eye as an indigo flower.

2. Now breathe in the indigo hue and see this being absorbed by the flower. Allow your imagination to create something that you want to manifest in your life.

3. Once you have completed this exercise take 3 deep breaths and open your eyes.

3 minute meditation for the Crown Chakra

1. Close your eyes and take 3 deep breaths as you exhale on the last breath bring your attention to the top of the head and imagine the Crown chakra as a pure white flower.

2. Now breathe in the white hue and see this being absorbed by the flower.

Imagine a column of white light connecting you to the source where you can receive pure energy. Visualize this light flowing all the way down through the chakras into the earth.

3. Once you have completed this exercise take 3 deep breaths and open your eyes.

Closing the Chakras

When the chakras have been opened to receive light and energy it is important that the petals are closed tightly before you participate in your daily routine.

3 easy steps for Closing the Chakras

1. Find yourself a comfortable place to either sit down with your feet on the floor or lie down with your hands by your side.

2. Now take 3 deep breaths as you inhale and exhale imagine starting at the top of your head and visualize the petals of the Crown chakra closing into a tight bud.

Repeat this process with all the chakras until you reach the Base chakra.

3. When you have completed this exercise you can then wrap yourself in a cloak of gold and silver light to seal in the positive energy.

Protection Meditation

Always protect yourself before and after all exercises by placing a cloak of gold and silver light around yourself as this will help to contain your positive energies. It is important that you protect yourself from other people's negative energy or if you ever feel tired and drained.

3 easy step for a Protection meditation

1. Find yourself a comfortable place to either sit down with your feet on the floor or lie down with your hands by your side.

2. Close your eyes and take 3 deep breaths as you inhale and exhale imagine that your body is being filled with a gold and silver light as it moves through your feet and into the earth. Repeat this 3 times.

Visualize a full length gold and silver cloak or a shield or an egg shaped bubble that covers your whole body.

Now, cover your head and feet and state 'I am always protected by the divine gold and silver light and I am safe and secure'.

3. When you have completed this exercise take 3 deep breaths and open your eyes.

Chapter Three

5 EASY STEP MEDITATION

When you have completed the 3 minute meditations and would like a more in-depth understanding of the chakras here are a few more meditations:-

5 easy step meditation for the Base Chakra

1. Find a quiet sacred place where you will not be interrupted and where you can sit comfortably with your feet on the ground.

2. Close your eyes and take 5 deep breaths as you exhale on the last breath bring your attention to the base of the spine and imagine your Base chakra as a deep ruby red crystal with 4 sides.

3. Now observe the colour, shape and texture of the ruby, notice if the crystal is chipped or discoloured.

4. If this ruby red crystal looks chipped in any way then you may take the time to heal this damage in whatever way you feel is appropriate.

If the crystal looks vibrant then you will know that your Base chakra is functioning properly.

5. When you have completed this exercise take another 5 deep breaths and open your eyes. You can visit your Base chakra at any time.

5 easy step meditation for the Sacral Chakra

1. Find a quiet sacred place where you will not be interrupted and where you can sit comfortably with your feet on the ground.

2. Close your eyes and take 5 deep breaths as you exhale on the last breath bring your attention to the area just below your navel and imagine that you see in front of you the ' fountain of life' representing your vitality.

Now, visualize your Sacral chakra as this fountain contains various shades of exotic orange flowers.

3. Observe the rate and speed of the fountain and see if it may need unblocking or cleaning. This will indicate if your Sacral chakra is healthy and functioning properly.

4. Now observe the colour, shape and texture of the flowers, notice if the flowers are healthy or unhealthy.

If any of the flowers look unhealthy then you may nurture and care for them in whatever way you feel is appropriate.

5. When you have completed this exercise take another 5 deep breaths and open your eyes. You can visit your Sacral chakra at anytime.

5 easy step meditation for the Solar Plexus

1. Find a quiet sacred place where you will not be interrupted and where you can sit or lie down whichever is the most comfortable position for you.

2. Close your eyes and take 5 deep breaths as you breathe out on the last breath bring your attention to a few inches above the navel.

Imagine a bright sun that is directly in front of you and bring the light from the sun allowing it to pass from the head area down into the Solar Plexus.

3. Now, observe the sun saturating your Solar Plexus with white positive light as the heat of the sun warms this area you will feel calm, peaceful, centred and in your own personal power.

Place a symbol of a triangle over the Solar Plexus as this will help to lock in the energy.

4. If you feel lethargic or a loss of energy in your Solar Plexus anytime throughout the day then you may breathe in to a count of 5 as you fill the Solar Plexus area with white positive light.

5. When you have completed this exercise take another 5 deep breaths and open your eyes.

Heart Meditation

5 easy step Diamond Crystal meditation

The diamond crystal meditation can be used to explore the many facets of love that you can experience.

When the diamond crystal is placed in the heart the eternal flame lights the darkness within and can be energized by day with the sun and by night with the moon.

1. Sit or lie down and breathe in 5 times then bring your attention to the centre of the chest area as you imagine the Heart chakra. Then observe the diamond crystal in the palm of your hand.

2. This diamond crystal represents the many facets of love that you can experience in your lifetime. Observe the crystalline structure and shape of the diamond in your hand.

3. Take the crystal and place this over the Heart chakra stating 'I now experience the many wonderful facets of love. I give and receive the love experience that is in total harmony and peace with everyone'.

Allow the crystal to merge and melt into your heart and acknowledge that you feel unconditional love, calmness and tranquility.

4. You will also observe that within the diamond there is the eternal flame that shines forth all light and love. This diamond crystal will light your way in any darkness or negative state and it can be energized by the sun in daylight and by the moon at night.

5. Now affirm 'I am a lovable and worthy person'. When you have completed this exercise take another 5 deep breaths and open your eyes.

The following meditation will support you in releasing any unresolved issues that may surface within the Heart chakra.

5 easy step meditation to release the negative patterns in the Heart Chakra

1. Sit or lie down and breathe in 5 times as you exhale on the last breath then imagine the Heart chakra as a large exotic pink flower with the petals tightly closed.

2. Notice the colour, shape, health and general condition of the flower as you gently open each petal individually.

3. Now cup your hands gently on either side of the flower and visualize a golden healing energy pouring into the flower causing the flower to change to a bright pink.

4. Take the pink flower and place this over the Heart chakra allowing it to merge and melt into the heart. Now, breathe deeply as you notice the pink energy in the Heart chakra turn to a green energy representing unconditional love.

At the same time acknowledge the part of yourself that may have any negative patterns or memories and let these hurt feelings arise allowing them to flow through the flower to be released.

5. Observe the memories and patterns being released and see them dissolve in the golden light and transmute into love.

Now affirm 'I am a lovable person and I deserve to have a wonderful loving soul to soul relationship'.

When you have completed this exercise take another 5 deep breaths and open your eyes.

5 easy step meditation for the Throat Chakra

1. Sit or lie down in a comfortable place as you close your eyes and take 5 deep breaths as you exhale on the last breath.

2. Bring your attention to the throat area breathing in as you visualize a blue lake that is pulsating with a blue light just in front of you.

3. Observe the texture of the water and notice if it is dull or vibrant. This will represent the state of your Throat chakra. If the water looks murky then your Throat chakra will need healing.

4. Imagine pouring an urn of clear water into the lake to purify and clean any debris as this will help you to express yourself and enhance your communication with others.

5. You can visit the clear blue lake that represents your throat chakra at any time to cleanse and purify.

When you have completed this exercise take another 5 deep breaths and open your eyes.

5 easy step meditation for the Third Eye Chakra

1. Sit or lie down and breathe in 5 times then bring your attention to the centre of the brow as you imagine the Third Eye and notice that you have a large amethyst crystal in the palm of your hand.

2. Observe the crystalline structure, shape and texture of the amethyst in your hand. Notice if the crystal is chipped or broken as this will reflect the state of the Third Eye chakra.

3. Now place the palm of your hand on the damaged areas of the amethyst crystal and observe it becoming perfect in shape. You may want to clean the crystal or replace some of the broken facets.

4. Take the crystal and place this over the Third eye stating 'I now experience the many dreams and visions that I am able create in my life'.

Allow the amethyst crystal to merge and melt into your Third eye and acknowledge that you are open to new visions and dreams to come to you.

You may focus on the new or full moon energy to assist you in manifesting your visions.

5. When you have completed this exercise take another 5 deep breaths and open your eyes.

5 easy step meditation for the Crown Chakra

1. Sit or lie down in a comfortable place as you close your eyes and take 5 deep breaths as you exhale on the last breath.

2. Bring your attention to the top of your head and visualize breathing in white light down into the Crown chakra and out through your feet.

3. Imagine that there are 5 white marble steps in front of you that lead to the 'temple of the lotus'. Begin walking up the white marble steps and observe if any steps are crumbling or broken or if they are in good condition.

This will indicate the well-being of your Crown chakra. You may repair any of the marble steps as you make your way towards the 'temple of the lotus'.

4. When you arrive at the fifth step you will notice the large thousand petal lotus flower that is in the middle of the temple with a blue flame that flickers from red to orange to yellow to green then blue to indigo.

Visualize this flame becoming a brilliant white light that pours from the lotus flower and illuminates the room bathing you all over.

If you feel depleted of energy or tired then you may replenish your energy from the 'temple of the lotus'.

5. When you have completed this meditation you may walk back down the steps and when you are ready take 5 deep breaths and open your eyes.

Chapter Four

SUNRISE MEDITATION

This is the Sunrise meditation that is similar to a wake-up call in the morning to help you to feel good and energize your body.

1. As you awake, notice that you feel relaxed from your dream state and take 7 deep breaths exhaling as you finish on the final breath.

2. Now, tune into your Base chakra and visualize a red vibrant colour pulsating and saturating the area. You then repeat this process with each chakra starting at the Sacral chakra (orange), followed by the Solar chakra (yellow), then the Heart chakra (green), Throat chakra (blue), Third eye chakra (indigo) and Crown chakra (white).

3. When you are at the Crown chakra you now visualize the white light cascading over your body and feel the vibrating new positive energy energizing your body. When you have completed this meditation take 7 deep breaths and open your eyes.

SUNSET MEDITATION

The Sunset meditation is a beautiful, soulful and harmonious meditation that can assist to restore your energy and tranquility.

It is a simple technique that aids the clearing of the chakras by breathing in the spectrum of the rainbow and releasing any negativity from the Aura.

1. Find a quiet sacred place where you will not be interrupted with your feet firmly on the ground. Close your eyes as you breathe 7 times and as you exhale on the last breath see in your mind's eye the Base chakra and breathe in the red hue.

2. As you breathe in this red shade also see yourself climbing steps or walking up a mountain to reach your destination. Now observe yourself standing on top of a mountain just in front of you is the beautiful sky and the lake and land below. It is important that you also see the horizon in the distance.

3. Now view the sun setting in the west as the deep red sun glows almost turning to an orange/yellow hue. This represents your Base chakra as you breathe in the red shade you are able to let go or release any negative issues.

4. Next focus your attention on the orange glow that surrounds the sun and breathe this vibrant colour 7 times into your Sacral chakra as you let go of any feelings of tiredness or exhaustion and then you can claim your creative energy.

5. Next focus on the yellow sun and breathe in and out 7 times into the Solar Plexus as you surrender the need to control and then you can claim your own power.

6. Now view the green fields and trees in the distance and look at the land as you connect to the Heart chakra. As you focus your attention on your breathing you are able to release any previous wounds or emotions as you exhale.

On the next intake of breath visualize unconditional love to the Heart chakra as you release your breath feel forgiveness and acceptance.

7. Observe the blue, purple and white streaks in the sunset. Next breathe the colour blue into your Throat chakra enhancing the voice area.

Envisage the purple streaks and white light and then breathe the purple streaks into the Third eye and the white light into the Crown chakra. As the sunset illuminates it bathes you in its glow and light connecting you to the higher divine consciousness and makes you feel at one.

8. From this position you are now part of a vibrating light that is pulsating this energy out like a beacon of light as you radiate the glorious rainbow spectrum state ' I am Magnificent'.

(go to step 10) ***Optional 9 only***

9. Now breathe 7 times and ask to see your soul's purpose in life only if you feel this is an appropriate time. You may ask for healing to release any blocks that stop you from moving forward. When you are ready and grounded you may put a Tetrahedron shape around your body to protect and seal in the energy.

10. When you feel totally safe and secure and grounded you can see yourself as a white light radiating out into the universe as a six pointed star. You are now the magnificent star of your own world reaching out into the universe beyond.

Next step 11 and 12

11. Next you may take 7 deep breaths starting at the crown as you breathe in the white light work your way downwards from the Crown chakra through the Third eye chakra, Throat chakra and into the Heart chakra asking for any blocks to be released as you breathe in unconditional love.

Next breathe into the Solar Plexus chakra, Sacral chakra and lastly the Base chakra breathing the red energy as you ground this energy into the crystalline structures into the earth.

12. When you are ready you may open your eyes. You will now feel full of a higher vibrational energy with all the wisdom, inspiration and calmness of spirit.

Afterword

<u>BASE CHAKRA</u>

Colour: Red

Located: Base of the Spine

Number of petals: 4

Element: Earth

Note: C

Gemstone: Red Jasper

Balanced: Ability to survive in a material world and bring ideas into action

Unbalanced: Angry, aggressive, and ungrounded

SACRAL CHAKRA

Colour: Orange

Located: few inches below the Navel

Number of petals: 6

Element: Water

Note: D

Gemstone: Carnelian

Balanced: Abundance of creative energy

Unbalanced: Low vitality and exhausted

SOLAR PLEXUS

Colour: Yellow

Located: above the Navel

Number of petals: 10

Element: Fire

Note: E

Gemstone: Calcite or Citrine

Balanced: Personal power and self-confidence

Unbalanced: Anxious and lacking in self-esteem

HEART CHAKRA

Colour: Green

Located: Chest area

Number of petals: 12

Element: Air

Note: F

Gemstone: Aventurine or Rose Quartz

Balanced: Compassion and unconditional love

Unbalanced: Control and manipulation

<u>THROAT CHAKRA</u>

Colour: Blue

Located: Throat area

Number of petals: 16

Element: Sound

Note: G

Gemstone: Sodalite or Sapphire

Balanced: Able to communicate and express oneself

Unbalanced: Unable to speak our truth with others

THIRD EYE CHAKRA

Colour: Indigo

Located: between the eyebrows

Number of petals: 2

Element: Light

Note: A

Gemstone: Lapis Lazuli

Balanced: Visions and dreams

Unbalanced: Unable to see clearly and lack imagination

CROWN CHAKRA

Colour: White

Located: Top of the head

Number of petals: 1000

Element: Thought

Note: B

Gemstone: Clear Quartz or Amethyst

Balance: Connect to the divine

Unbalance: Depressed and isolated

SOUL II SOUL

My love for you is as constant as the sun that rises in the East and sets in the West as everlasting as the eons of time that may separate us.

My need for you is like the fire that burns passionately in the hearth smouldering to a glowing ember.

My need for you is as solid as the ground beneath my feet with landscape that will never change no matter where you are.

My need for you is the cool breeze on the ocean surface.

My need for you is the ebbing and flowing of the waves on the sea shore and the eternal love of the sunlight that dances on the surface of the sea.

My need for you is like the water as it soaks your skin and caresses your soul.

When night falls my love for you will shine brightly as the Evening Star.

My love for you is like the Morning Star as it lights your way in the darkness and guides you in life's journey to a new day.